The Life of

Florence Sabin

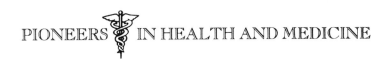

PIONEERS IN HEALTH AND MEDICINE

The Life of

Florence Sabin

Judith Kaye

Twenty-First Century Books

A Division of Henry Holt and Company

New York

PHOTO CREDITS
pages 6, 16, and 34: Sophia Smith Collection, Smith College. **pages 48, and 56:** UPI/Bettmann. **pages 68, 73, and 77:** Sophia Smith Collection, Smith College.

Twenty-First Century Books
A Division of Henry Holt and Company, Inc.
115 West 18th Street
New York, NY 10011

Library of Congress Cataloging-in-Publication Data

Kaye, Judith
The Life of Florence Sabin / Judith Kaye. — 1st ed.
p. cm. — (Pioneers in Health and Medicine)
Includes biographical references and index.
Summary: A biography of the physician who made significant contributions to the field of medicine as a researcher, professor, and public health advocate and who became the first woman ever to be elected to the National Academy of Sciences.
1. Sabin, Florence Rena, 1871–1953. 2. Immunologists—United States—Biography—Juvenile literature. 3. Women physicians—United States—Biography—Juvenile literature. [1. Sabin, Florence Rena, 1871–1953. 2. Women physicians. 3. Physicians.]
I. Title. II. Series.
QR180.72.S23K38 1993
616.079'092--dc20 [B] 92–34419 CIP AC

ISBN 0–8050–2299–6
First Edition—1993

Printed in Mexico
All first editions are printed on acid-free paper ∞.

10 9 8 7 6 5 4 3 2 1

9312246

Contents

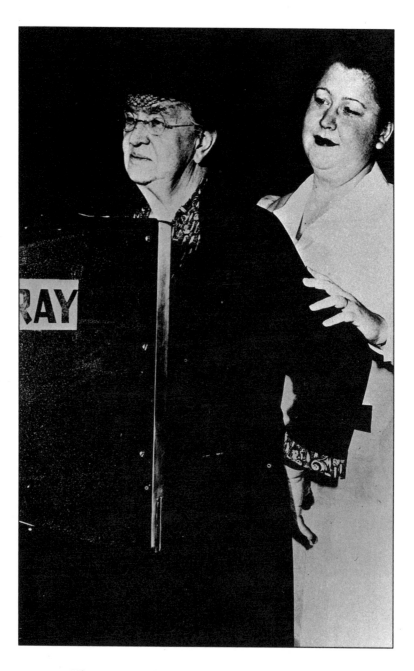

Florence Sabin having an x-ray taken

1

Advocate for Colorado's Health

On a crowded street in downtown Denver, Colorado, a seventy-eight-year-old woman stood next to a small, makeshift hut. The hut was marked with a sign that read "x-ray." The year was 1951.

The woman smiled as she stood before two newspaper photographers. The photographers clicked their shutters as their subject fidgeted impatiently.

The sturdy, gray-haired woman, her brown eyes glowing behind thick glasses, was Florence Rena Sabin. She was recognized by many as the foremost woman scientist of her time. As manager of Denver's health department, Dr. Sabin was launching a campaign to provide free chest x-rays. Throughout the day, people would stop by the booth for a quick x-ray. Sabin hoped that the free program would help diagnose cases of the fatal lung disease tuberculosis in its early stages.

So far, the x-ray program had served hundreds of thousands of people. Of those, 4,243 were found to have tuberculosis, which is curable if caught in time. Once the disease was detected, these people could be helped, perhaps saving their lives.

Sabin, who had created this life-saving program, could have stayed in her office while the x-rays were taken. Instead, she worked in the booths with the other volunteers. Sabin was determined to make the program work.

Determination defined Florence Sabin's personality. In the early 1900s, when Sabin began her career, women who wished to work as doctors and scientists faced many obstacles. With quiet perseverance, Sabin overcame prejudice to become the first woman to head a department at Johns Hopkins Medical School. Later, she was the first woman appointed as a member of the Rockefeller Institute for Medical Research in New York City. There, she led a team conducting research on several important topics, including the causes of tuberculosis. Perhaps Florence Sabin's greatest honor was her election as the first woman member of the National Academy of Sciences.

Dr. Sabin believed that effort and ability would overcome discrimination. "Women," she once said, "can have whatever they are willing to work for."

In spite of her brilliant research career, Florence Sabin certainly wasn't used to having her picture taken by reporters. Anyone who had known her as a medical researcher who loved the order of her laboratory might have been surprised to see her as a crusading public health officer. Florence might have been surprised herself.

As a professor and researcher, Sabin had lived quietly. Her life had focused on her laboratory studies and her students. Eleven years earlier, after more than forty years of teaching and peering through microscopes, she had returned to her native Colorado for a peaceful retirement.

But her retirement hadn't lasted long. She launched a new career at age seventy-three, when the governor of Colorado appointed her to head the health committee of a state planning commission.

Dr. Sabin plunged enthusiastically into the task of improving health conditions for the people of Colorado. She was eager to meet the challenge of a new kind of medical work—public health.

Public health work involves public action— determining the effects of policies, laws, and practices on the health of the general public, and developing new policies, laws, and practices to improve that health. If people are becoming sick from contaminated water, a private physician treats them, one by one, for their illnesses. A public health doctor, on the other hand, tries to locate the source of contamination and works to have the water supply purified.

In a sense, Florence Sabin had always been involved in public health. As a researcher, she had contributed to a greater understanding of the cells in the body. Eventually, a better understanding of how human cells function was to aid researchers in finding cures for diseases like tuberculosis, diseases that caused millions of deaths each year.

Sabin began her investigation of Colorado's health system just as she might have begun a laboratory experiment, with background research into the problem. In order to learn about and to evaluate health conditions, she had two doctors conduct a survey. The survey found that Colorado had some of the worst health conditions in the country.

Dr. Sabin was shocked. "We think of our state as a health resort," she said, "yet we're dying faster than people in most states."

Sabin learned that many people were becoming seriously ill after eating meat from sick cattle, for almost half the state's cattle were infected with disease. Milk supplies were also unhealthy. In one town, Dr. Sabin reported, "the women said that they could see so much dirt in the milk that they did not use it at all." In many parts of the state, the drinking water posed a threat to people's health. Many communities lacked good sewage treatment, and the water supplies were dangerously polluted as a result.

In addition, vegetables that had been fertilized with manure from sick cattle and irrigated with polluted water were not safe to eat. The vegetables were so unhealthy some Colorado restaurants posted signs to attract customers. The signs read, "No Colorado Vegetables Served Here."

People from other states often came to Colorado's Rocky Mountains to recover from tuberculosis. Yet many of Colorado's own citizens were dying from tuberculosis each year. And there were not enough hospital beds for Coloradans suffering from tuberculosis and other serious diseases. Between 1940 and 1945, due to poor care and unhealthy conditions, more than 14,000 people in Colorado had died from diseases that could have been prevented or controlled. Florence Sabin calculated that 8,245 of these people could have been saved. During these same five years, many Americans had been killed fighting World War II in Europe and the Pacific. But Colorado's health conditions were so poor that the state had lost more citizens who died needlessly from controllable diseases than it had lost soldiers who died on the battlefields of World War II.

Sabin fought back by convincing politicians to introduce a series of bills that would address the state's health problems. The bills called for several reforms requiring better standards for milk and beef. They called for measures to clean up the water that was contaminating food supplies. The bills would force Colorado to organize its health department more efficiently and to allocate more money for hospitals and other health facilities.

To insure that the bills got proper attention, Dr. Sabin crisscrossed the state, giving speeches to groups of citizens in hundreds of small towns. The people of Colorado deserved "health to match our mountains," she told them. Her goal was to make people care enough about the health problems in their state that they would force their elected politicians to pay attention.

The story of an elderly woman doctor journeying through mountain snowstorms to fight for health reforms drew the attention of local newspapers and magazines throughout Colorado. One article described Sabin's convincing campaign:

> *There was a little bump of a woman with a twinkly sort of smile that made her eyeglasses seem to light up. She started to talk. . .before I knew it I had promised to work on her committee.*

Praising Dr. Sabin's efforts, a public health official called her "a lovable volcano." Florence Sabin was becoming a well-known personality. All over Colorado, people were growing indignant about Colorado's poor health conditions. Politicians could no longer ignore the issues she presented.

By 1947, most of the Sabin bills had passed and become law. But Sabin still wasn't ready to retire. She began to focus her energy on the programs for the city of Denver, which was exempt from state laws. Denver was where she instituted the free x-ray campaign. Following that program, the tuberculosis rate in Denver was cut in half. Dr. Sabin was keeping her promise to eliminate unnecessary deaths in Colorado. "If even one child's life may be saved," she told those who criticized the cost of health programs, "is that not enough?"

Once, Florence Sabin expressed a vision of "a time. . .when men and women will live their allotted span quietly, without illness, free from pain." She hoped a time would come when all diseases could be prevented or cured. First as a researcher, and later as an advocate for public health, she tried to make this vision real.

2

Family Ties

Florence Sabin's grandmother once told her that doctors "ran in the family." In 1798, Levi Sabin had been the first Sabin who was doctor. Florence's Uncle Robert was a physician. Her own father, George, had almost become a doctor. But in 1859, when he heard promising stories of discoveries of gold in Colorado, George Sabin changed his mind and headed west.

In those days, leaving the cities and towns of the East meant leaving civilization behind. George Sabin traveled by stagecoach. His two thousand-mile journey took him over the Appalachian mountains and through the vast stretches of the Great Plains. He traveled six hundred miles across the plains on roads that were little more than ruts caused by wagon wheels of other travelers. He encountered few settlements of any type. The stagecoach passengers faced the threat of becoming lost, running out of food, or being attacked by Indians.

When he reached Colorado in 1860, George Sabin discovered that mining for gold was not going to make him rich immediately. But he decided to stay and try to make a career as a miner. He spent long weeks at mountain camps digging for gold. Eventually, George settled in Central City, Colorado. The small town had developed in the mountains to serve the miners who were clustered there.

The Colorado gold rush also brought Florence's mother, Rena Sabin, to the West. Although Rena was from Vermont, she was teaching in Georgia during the Civil War. When General Sherman led Union forces on a destructive march through Georgia, burning cities and ruining farms, the state was devastated.

Rena saw a newspaper ad seeking a teacher for a small Colorado mining town, and she seized the opportunity to leave the turmoil and fighting behind. She journeyed by stagecoach to Black Hawk, a town not far from where George Sabin lived. Rena and George met at a dance, and a month later they decided to marry.

The Sabins' first child, Mary, was born in 1869. Florence was born two years later, on November 9, 1871. During the early years of Florence's life, the family lived in a small, comfortable two-story frame house in Central City.

By the 1870s, Central City was a bustling town nestled in Colorado's Rocky Mountains. What little is

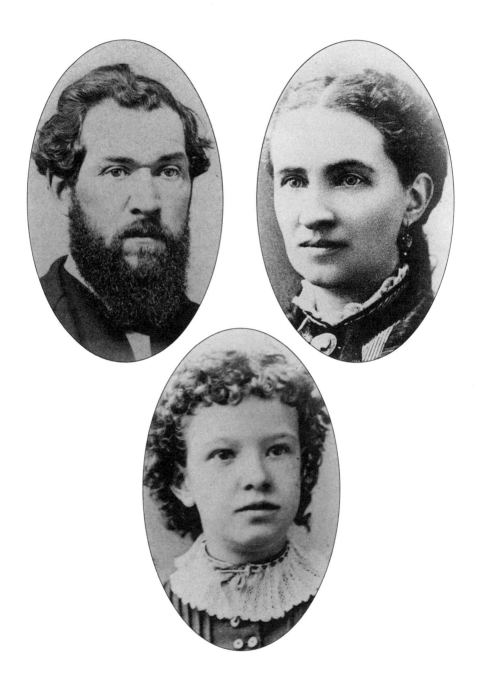

George, Rena, and Florence Sabin

known of Florence's early years there was recorded by her sister, Mary. Mary described their house:

> *Steps led to a porch and the front door opened into the dining room. Opposite the door was a stairway to the second floor. At the head of the stairs a door opened to a short bridge to the back yard, for the first floor stood against a vertical wall of solid stone.*

The Sabins' home and lifestyle were typical of that of many miner families. They kept two horses for transportation, and a cow to provide milk. Central City had no water supply, so tanks of water were brought in by horse and wagon. As Mary wrote, "Water was peddled from door to door by a man atop a big tank wagon, who charged 50 cents a barrel for his precious cargo, which he delivered through a hose." The water was stored in two large vats inside the house. As an adult, Florence looked back on this water-delivery system with horror. She realized that the water must have been terribly impure.

By modern standards, health conditions in the mining town were terrible. In the nineteenth century, health care practices were still primitive, and—especially in the newly settled western territories—medical care was often inaccessible or inadequate. In addition, the importance of cleanliness, or sanitation, in preventing the spread of disease was not yet understood. Unclean water and foods often produced sickness. Very little was known of what caused or cured illnesses, and diseases that are now easily preventable then led to early deaths. Many babies died in infancy, and mothers often suffered fatal complications during childbirth.

In spite of these conditions, Florence and Mary were healthy, energetic children. Often, they helped their mother. Across from their house, a steep path led to the Fred Kruse grocery store, to which Florence and Mary ran errands for their mother. They had to be careful on the narrow road. Once, a mule team with a load of gold ore almost ran over Florence. Just in time, Mary shoved her out of the way.

When they weren't busy with chores, Florence and Mary roamed the hillsides near their home. They liked to look for birds and collect wild flowers.

The sisters also enjoyed singing in the parlor with their parents. George and Rena Sabin were delighted that the girls had a liking for music. They knew that music was an important part of a well-rounded education, and they intended to provide their daughters with the best education possible.

In 1875, George Sabin purchased a small mining company and moved his family to Denver. The Sabins welcomed the move, for the schools in Denver were much better than those near Central City, and Mary would soon enter the first grade.

Florence never forgot the day that she and her mother walked Mary to her first day of school. Four-year-old Florence saw some children drinking water from a dipper that they filled from an old wooden bucket. She was thirsty, and she asked her mother if she could have some of the water. But Rena said no. Her mother told her that she should never drink from anyone else's cup. Florence would have to wait until she got home and could use her own clean cup. More than seventy years later, when Florence was working to clean up Colorado's water supply, she referred to this incident as "my first lesson in good public-health practices."

After Mary started spending her days in school, Florence, who had few friends other than her sister, grew lonely and bored. When her mother gave birth to a baby boy, Richman, Florence was delighted. She cherished the little boy and spent many happy hours helping her mother care for him. But Richman died in 1877. His death left Florence bewildered and frightened.

The following year, Rena gave birth to a second son, Albert. Florence was happy to have another baby in the house. But her joy was short-lived. Rena did not recover from this birth. She remained weak and was often ill until she finally died—on Florence's seventh birthday. Florence was tremendously upset. Later she called the day on which her mother died the last day of her childhood.

The death of his wife left a sorrowful George Sabin with three children to care for while he worked long, hard days in the mine to support his family. Realizing that he could not manage by himself, George sent little Albert to live with the children's Aunt Min in Central City, and the still-grieving Florence and Mary to Wolfe Hall, a local boarding school. From that time on, Florence and Mary were moved from home to home and from school to school. And, although the adults in Florence's family were warm and loving, her sister, Mary, was her only constant companion. Shy Florence became very dependent on the more outgoing Mary, and they remained close throughout their lives.

During their stay at Wolfe Hall, the sisters often dreamed of ways to reunite their family. But all their hopes shattered when they learned that little Albert, too, had died, shortly after his first birthday. Much later, Mary remembered telling Florence, "There's no one left except Papa and us. He'll stay up there at the mine and we'll live in Wolfe Hall till we die."

The summer after sending them to Wolfe Hall, George Sabin invited his daughters to visit him at the mining camp of Leadville. Leadville, sometimes called Cloud City, was located among broad hillsides and jagged peaks high in the Rockies. But the camp itself was bleak and barren. The streets were always dusty or muddy, depending on weather, and the miners lived in drab, dirty boardinghouses with leaky roofs.

At first, Florence was shy and withdrawn. She was intimidated by the rough miners, and she resented George Sabin for abandoning her at Wolfe Hall. But soon her father won back her affections. He had bought her a special red raincoat and boots and a hard hat, so that she could go into the mine. Florence enjoyed riding in an ore bucket down a mine shaft into the damp depths.

George Sabin understood that his daughters, who were then eleven and nine years old, needed a home. He arranged for them to live with his brother Albert's family in Lake Forest, Illinois, near Chicago. "We'll be in a home again," Florence rejoiced when the girls received the news. "We'll be part of a family!"

The sisters made the move happily and settled in comfortably with their uncle's family. Uncle Albert and his wife seemed pleased to have more children living with them and their son, Stewart. They provided Florence with the security that she so needed in her life.

Although Uncle Albert loved the girls, he was always careful not to become a replacement for George Sabin. He gently reminded Florence that he only had her "on loan," and that her real home was still with her father in Colorado.

Living with the Albert Sabin family rekindled

Florence's interest in music, for music was an important part of the family's life. "Aunty is playing on the piano," Florence wrote in a letter to her father, "and it sounds lovely." During the family sings, in which Florence and Mary joined readily, eleven-year-old Stewart usually played the piano. When Florence expressed interest in learning to play, Uncle Albert encouraged her to start taking piano lessons.

In 1881, Albert took Stewart and his nieces to visit their grandparents in Saxtons River, Vermont, the state in which both George and Rena Sabin had grown up. Florence and Mary discovered a natural environment of lakes, streams, and dark green forests very different from any they had seen before. The gently rounded Vermont mountains contrasted with the sharp peaks of the Colorado Rockies. And what a change it was to see neatly painted farmhouses, instead of crude mining camps, nestled in the valleys.

Florence loved to hear her Grandmother Sabin tell about family history. It was their grandmother who told the girls about the doctors in the family. Grandmother Sabin must have thought that Florence had the makings of a doctor herself. "Too bad you're not a boy," she told her granddaughter. "You would have made a good doctor." Like most people in the late 1800s, Grandmother Sabin believed that practicing medicine was a man's profession.

Two years later, shortly before Florence's twelfth

birthday, the sisters returned to Saxtons River to attend the Vermont Academy, a school with an excellent reputation. The girls lived with their grandmother and grandfather in an old, white farmhouse. They spent many evenings listening to their grandparents tell stories about their father. Florence missed him very much. "When I'm through school, I'm going back to Colorado and make a home for Papa," she confided to Mary. "He shouldn't be living in boarding-houses all alone."

Unfortunately, Grandmother Sabin died during the girls' first winter in Vermont, and they went back to Illinois. There Florence resumed her piano lessons and began to think seriously about becoming a professional pianist. Later that year, when Mary decided to return to school in Vermont, Florence joined her sister at the Vermont Academy.

When Mary graduated from the Academy, she enrolled in Smith College, one of the first American colleges for women. With Mary away at school in Massachusetts, Florence felt somewhat lost. She spent the following year in the security of her uncle's home, where she continued to practice the piano. However, at the urging of Uncle Albert, she returned to the Vermont Academy the next year to complete her studies. Her uncle had bought her a piano to keep at school, and she practiced tirelessly.

One day, while Florence was repeating a series of

piano exercises, another student complained that she was tired of hearing the same drills over and over. She begged Florence to play a waltz or a march. Florence replied that she must practice the exercises "because I intend to make music my career."

Annoyed, the other girl told Florence she wasn't good enough to be a professional, and that she would never be more than an ordinary musician, no matter how hard she worked. The remark stung. But, stubbornly, Florence continued her practice to the end. Then she closed the piano lid and went off to think.

Despite her love for music, Florence suspected that the girl was right—she would never be a great pianist. If so, Florence decided, she certainly could never settle for being an average musician. Whatever her career, Florence wanted to be the best. She decided to give up music and focus her energy on academic subjects.

Determined to graduate with honors, Florence switched to the most difficult classes, the college preparatory courses. She put the energy she had devoted to her music into studying science textbooks and preparing laboratory experiments.

Florence's determined scholarship did not go unnoticed. In 1889, she was elected president of her graduating class. As she went through the graduation ceremony, she was proud of her accomplishments. She looked forward to the fall, when she would join her sister at Smith College.

3

School Days

The idea of a college for women was a new one when Smith College first opened in 1875. By the time Florence came to the school, fourteen years later, Smith had developed strong academic programs.

Florence was eighteen years old when she arrived at Smith. The short young woman had frizzy hair. She could hardly see a thing without the glasses on her nose. In spite of her academic success, Florence was still very shy. She must have been relieved that Mary, now in her third year, had arranged for her sister to have a room in the same boardinghouse.

Florence studied hard at Smith, where she decided to major in science. She received high grades in zoology, biology, chemistry, and geology. In her sophomore year, she studied with John Tappan Stoddard, head of the department of chemistry. Professor Stoddard encouraged Florence's interest in scientific investigation. He emphasized the importance of "learning to reason logically from observed facts to a conclusion." Although he explained basic theories and laws during his lectures, he encouraged his students to make their own observations and form their own judgments about what they saw.

Even outside of the classroom, Florence's activities revolved around her new interest in scientific investigation. She was invited to join the Colloquium, a small discussion group that met on a regular basis with Professor Stoddard. Although the group's discussions usually focused on scientific subjects, the members of the Colloquium had fun, too. Sometimes they held "chemical tea parties," using laboratory equipment to mix and serve their tea.

While Florence enjoyed her college years, she sometimes worried about her future. What would she do after she graduated from Smith? In the 1890s, most women married when they finished their educations, if not before. Few thought of having a career. But Florence wasn't sure she would ever get married.

In her junior year, after Mary had graduated and gone back to Denver to teach mathematics, Florence became even more concerned about her future. She was lonely without her sister. She wondered what the rest of her life would be like.

One Saturday night, when most of the students were at a party, Florence made a decision. She decided to begin planning a career. She thought about her passion for science. She remembered her grandmother's talk about doctors in the family. Perhaps she should become a doctor, Florence thought.

Florence decided to talk with Dr. Grace Preston, the school doctor at Smith, who lived in the same boardinghouse and who had encouraged Florence in her studies.

Dr. Preston spoke with Florence at length about the difficulties women faced in becoming doctors. The first woman to graduate from medical school in the United States was Elizabeth Blackwell, who received her degree in 1849. She had faced much opposition and had been rejected by many medical schools before finally being accepted by Geneva College.

In the forty years that followed Blackwell's graduation, more women entered the medical profession. In fact, in the nineteenth century, medicine attracted more American women than any other profession except teaching. By the 1890s, there were several thousand women doctors. Although relatively few women were accepted by medical schools, several medical colleges exclusively for women had been established over the years. But even after they received training, women faced discrimination. Female doctors were often viewed as less competent than male doctors. They rarely received the respect and recognition that they deserved.

Florence listened to Dr. Preston's stories. But she

wasn't discouraged. She had decided to become a doctor.

Florence Sabin was fortunate in her timing. Unlike many women before her, she did not have to face the struggle of gaining admittance to a "men's" medical school. The Johns Hopkins University, first opened in 1876, had established a hospital in 1887, after the Quaker merchant, Johns Hopkins, had left his fortune "for the care of the indigent sick poor of Baltimore." Now there was to be a new medical school, as well, and both men and women were to be admitted.

"The opening of the Johns Hopkins Medical School in 1893 was made possible by a fund raised by a group of women," Florence later explained. And, according to Sabin, "far more important than the actual gift of money, which determined the time of opening the new medical school, were the conditions under which the fund was given and accepted." In exchange for their gift of money, the women, joined in an organization named the Women's Committee, insisted upon "the admission of women on the same terms as men." The Women's Committee also required that entering students have "a college degree or its equivalent, a knowledge of physics, chemistry and biology, and proficiency in foreign languages."

In those days, the quality of medical schools in the United States varied. There were very few requirements for entering students. The most ambitious Americans went to European medical schools for training, because the European schools were better. The Baltimore Women's Committee hoped to make Johns Hopkins a model for modern medical schools.

Florence was very excited to learn about Johns Hopkins. With her Smith education, she could meet the admission requirements. But Florence would not be able to enter the first class at the medical school. She could not afford the tuition. On a visit to Denver, Florence told Mary that she wanted to study medicine. Mary explained that their father's mining company was not doing well enough to pay for medical school tuition.

So Florence launched a fund-raising effort of her own. To earn the money she needed, Florence worked for three years after graduating from Smith College. The first year she taught at Wolfe Hall, the Denver boarding school she and Mary had attended after the death of their mother. Florence spent the following summer in Wisconsin, teaching science to the children of a wealthy doctor.

This job proved to be an exciting experience. She taught the children by letting them touch, see, and explore nature's wonders for themselves. Her self-confidence soared as she witnessed the success of her teaching methods. And she developed a life-long friendship with the family, the Denisons.

Florence returned to Denver to teach at Wolfe Hall for a second year. The following year, she was lucky enough to get a teaching position at Smith College, her alma mater. By 1896 Florence had saved enough money for medical school. She was almost twenty-five years old when she entered Johns Hopkins Medical School.

Florence Sabin's medical education at Johns Hopkins took four years. During the first year, students learned about the normal functioning of the healthy human body. Sabin particularly liked anatomy, the study of the structure of animals and plants, and histology, in which she studied the structure of cells. These classes weren't mere lectures. By examining thin slices of human tissue under a microscope, students made their own discoveries about the arrangement and function of systems in the human body.

The second year Sabin studied the diseased body. She learned what occurred in the body's cells and organs when a person became sick. She learned how diseases were spread through microscopic organisms called germs, a relatively new discovery at the time. She became familiar with the drugs that were available. But she didn't see any patients yet. When she studied surgery, the operations were performed on live, anesthetized animals.

In the third year, Sabin and her classmates put on white coats, hung stethoscopes around their necks, and moved from their labs into clinics, where they worked with real patients. At the Hopkins hospital dispensary, or clinic, the poor paid fifteen cents, if they could; those who could not pay were treated free.

During their final year, Sabin's class was divided into four sections, or groups. The groups rotated, concentrating for two months on each of the following subjects: surgery; medicine; obstetrics, which deals with pregnancy and childbirth; and gynecology, the branch of medicine that focuses on issues of health specific to women.

While women may have been admitted to Johns Hopkins on the same basis as men, that did not mean the men and women students were treated equally. The fifteen women in Sabin's class of forty-two roomed together in a dormitory known as the "Hen House," and they were sometimes insultingly referred to as "Hen Medics." Some male students went out of their way to tease the women, and some teachers made it clear that they regarded the female students as inferior to male students.

Sabin tried to ignore such treatment. She continued to do the best work she could. She felt her job was to keep studying, and not to worry about the men's jokes and insults.

At Johns Hopkins, students were encouraged to do investigative research on their own. Once again,

Florence's excellent work drew the attention of a teacher, Dr. Franklin Paine Mall.

Mall, the school's first professor of anatomy, had studied under several famous scientists in Germany. His teachers there had convinced him that students learned best when they had the chance to make discoveries on their own. Sabin later described Mall's low-key method of teaching:

> He never gave first-hand praise; the only encouragement which a student received was a genuine interest in his work shown in such a way that the student came to find enjoyment where Dr. Mall found his—in the work itself.

Mall's philosophy of teaching was to present his students with a question or a problem and to let the students find the answer with little or no guidance. He had a sign posted in his anatomy laboratory: "Your Body Is Your Textbook." Many years later, Florence joked about Mall's method by claiming that when the doctor watched his wife give their baby a bath, he asked, "Why don't you just put her in the water and let her work out her own technique?"

Mall liked to give his best students extra projects on which to work, and he soon had extra work for Florence. She was content to spend long hours in the lab, learning through investigation. Dr. Mall was very impressed by the research Florence did on the nervous system, the network of nerve cells and nervous tissue in the body. He encouraged Florence to publish her first academic paper, a high honor for a student.

When the paper was accepted for publication, Florence proudly sent off a copy to her father and another to Uncle Albert Sabin. She never learned of her father's reaction—he died before he could answer her letter. However, Albert Sabin, who supported Florence in all her endeavors, wrote back that, no matter what the outcome of her research, now or in the future, "your old Uncle will love you still and believe you are the best of the pack."

In Florence's senior year, Dr. Mall asked her to study the structure of the brain of newborn infants. He provided her with several slides of tissue from a newborn's brain, which she examined closely under the microscope. Sabin made useful and unexpected discoveries about the structure of the lower part of the brain, and she used her observations to build a model showing the structure of the newborn's lower brain. Copies of Sabin's model were used in medical schools for many years. In 1901, the year after she graduated, Florence published this research as *An Atlas of the Medulla and Midbrain*, which would become a classic text on the subject.

Although Florence felt at home in the lab, during her senior year she spent most of her time in the hospital. The atmosphere there was much more hectic

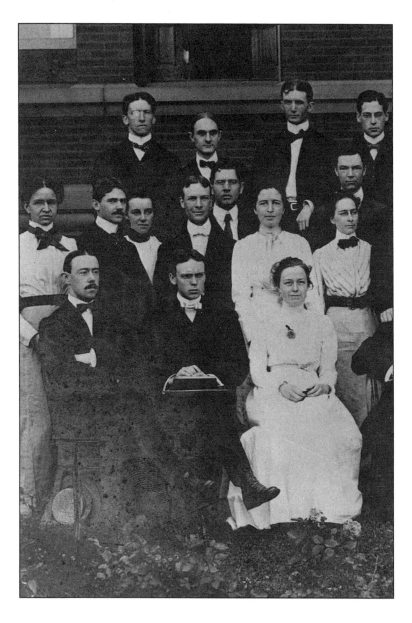

Florence Sabin (second row left) and part of her medical school class, including Dorothy Reed (same row, last on right)

than in the calm laboratory. In one two-month period, when Florence worked in obstetrics, she delivered nine babies and was on call twenty-four hours a day until those nine babies were born. During this time, Sabin slept with her clothes laid out on a chair, ready to be pulled on, for she never knew when she would be called to a pregnant woman's home. When the call came, she would rush to the woman's bedside. There, under conditions that were often crowded and unsanitary, she would deliver the child and help the mother through the birth.

Florence was relieved when these two months were over. She had learned more from her work in obstetrics than just how to deliver babies. She had learned a lesson about herself. "I don't seem to work well under pressure," she wrote in a letter to Mary. "I need a calm and placid atmosphere." She liked to have the time to perform each task perfectly, to check her work, and to repeat a task if necessary. In the laboratory environment, she had that time. Florence realized that she was more interested in research than in working directly with patients.

As she neared the end of her senior year of medical school, Florence needed to select an area of medicine in which to specialize. It was not a difficult decision. After her experience in obstetrics, she was able to select her specialty—medical research—with ease. As a researcher, Florence could work in the controlled laboratory setting she preferred.

But first, after she graduated from medical school in 1900, Florence needed to complete her education by serving as an intern, or assistant physician, on a hospital staff. The openings for interns at Johns Hopkins Hospital were awarded to the top students in the class. Florence Sabin, as the third best student in her class, and Dorothy Reed, as the fourth, were in line for two of these internships.

However, the hospital authorities soon made it clear that they intended to grant only one of the internships to a woman. For the first time, Florence faced the possibility of being denied a position she had earned, simply because she was a woman. This discrimination made her very uneasy. Her reaction was to withdraw from the competition altogether. She told Dorothy Reed that she would accept, instead, a research fellowship that had been offered to her.

By backing out, Florence intended to clear the way for Reed to accept the one "woman's" internship available, and to avoid an uncomfortable confrontation. But Reed refused to give in to antifeminist thinking.

"We both go, or forget it," she told Sabin. Reed's determination convinced Sabin to hold firm, and both women eventually got the internships they deserved.

4

"Pass It On"

The internship year proved difficult for Florence Sabin. Her supervisor at the hospital did not believe that women should be doctors, and he treated her badly. As usual, Sabin tried to ignore the treatment and go about her business, determined to let her good work speak for her.

At one point an exasperated Dorothy Reed blurted out, "I simply cannot understand how you can take such treatment without fighting back."

"I just don't like scenes, that's all," Sabin calmly replied. "I'm doing my work, so what does it matter?"

When the year was over, Sabin happily accepted a research position in Dr. Mall's laboratory. The Baltimore Women's Committee, which followed the careers of all women medical students at Johns Hopkins with interest, was impressed with her success. The committee provided her with a fellowship of seventy-five dollars a month.

Dr. Mall assigned Sabin a research project on the formation of the lymphatic system, which consists of tiny vessels branching throughout the entire body. Today we know that the lymph vessels carry lymph fluid, which contains nutrients from the blood. The lymphatic system distributes these materials from the blood throughout the body.

In the early 1900s, however, the lymphatic system was not well understood. Scientists believed the lymph vessels were completely separate from the blood vessels. They designed many experiments to determine exactly how the lymphatic system worked and what it looked like.

Sabin's task was to attempt to trace the development of the lymphatic system in an unborn animal. She worked by injecting dyes into lymph fluid taken from tissues of unborn pigs. Under a microscope, the colored dyes allowed her to see how the lymph fluid flowed through the lymphatic system.

Sabin discovered that the lymphatic vessels were not separate from the blood vessels, as had been previously thought. Instead, she found, lymph vessels grew like buds out of blood vessels that had already developed in the unborn animal.

Sabin's discovery was significant to the understanding of the lymphatic system. The scientific community was surprised to learn of a connection between the blood vessels and the lymphatic system.

At first, not everyone was convinced by Sabin's research. But as more scientists examined her work, they realized her observations were accurate.

Florence Sabin's work was published in the *American Journal of Anatomy* in 1902. In the spring of that year, Sabin's fellowship in Dr. Mall's lab expired. Her research had been so outstanding that the Johns Hopkins Medical School offered her an assistant professorship in anatomy. Sabin was thrilled. The research and teaching position was exactly what she wanted. It would allow her to continue working with Professor Mall. And she was happy to stay in Baltimore. She had grown fond of the city's narrow streets, alleys, and row houses.

In 1903, Sabin received the Naples Table Association Prize of $1,000. This fellowship had been established by a group of American women who wanted to encourage other women to study at a famous research facility in Naples, Italy. Slowly, Sabin was earning wider recognition for her research ability.

For the next twenty-three years, Sabin spent most of her time at the medical school. The red-brick building was situated in East Baltimore, the dirtiest and most unattractive part of the city, near a busy railway station. But the school's laboratories were light and cheerful, and once inside their bright yellow walls, Sabin felt totally at home.

She soon felt at home in the classroom as well.

Although her lectures were a bit stiff and formal in the beginning, as the years went by, Florence Sabin grew more confident of her teaching. Her shyness slowly faded, and she gained a reputation as a compelling lecturer. Her presentations were never repetitious. After giving a lecture, she tore up her notes, forcing herself to think the subject through anew the following year. She used fresh thoughts, words, and examples. Her introductory anatomy lectures were famous—students who were not studying anatomy, and even other staff members, often stopped in to listen.

Dr. Sabin had learned her teaching methods from Dr. Mall. Like Mall, she assigned students laboratory problems and then left them to learn from their own mistakes and discoveries. Mall had taught her that she should "never make the directions so specific as to rob the student of his pleasure in discovery and make him mechanically follow a definite procedure."

Sometimes, though, it was hard for Dr. Sabin not to get involved. "One of my most vivid memories," a student later recalled, "is of her sitting beside me as I looked through a microscope at a histological preparation. She cared so much about my seeing the important points on the slide that she all but lent me eyes for the occasion."

Florence Sabin was very popular with her students. She had adopted Dr. Mall's motto, "Pass it on," and, like Mall, she became mentor to many promising students. She pushed her students to do difficult and original research.

During her years at Johns Hopkins, Sabin herself kept extremely busy. When she wasn't teaching, she continued her independent research. For her, research combined well with teaching. "All teachers should be engaged in research," she said. "Research lifts teaching to a higher plane." She firmly believed that "the class can be taught in the spirit of research, which means that it is more important for the student to be able to find out something for himself than to memorize what someone else has said."

Dr. Sabin always managed to squeeze in time to spend in her laboratory, whether it was between classes, early in the morning, or late at night. Knowing how important the research was to her, students made a point of tiptoeing past Sabin's lab so they wouldn't break her concentration.

Between 1902 and 1911, Sabin's research centered on the lymphatic system. She published several more papers on the subject, culminating her studies in "The Development of the Lymphatic System." This paper became an important chapter in a textbook titled *Manual of Human Embryology*.

Once her research on the lymphatic system was complete, Florence Sabin turned to studying the blood vessels themselves, and how they formed in an unborn animal. On a visit to the University of Leipzig in Germany, she had learned a new technique for staining live cells, injecting the cells with dye so their movements through the circulatory system could be traced. With the new technique, Sabin was able to watch changes in live tissue, rather than in inactive dead tissue, under her microscope.

Dr. Sabin probably used this new technique one night when she stayed up till dawn, alone in her laboratory, examining a live chick embryo. During what she called "the most exciting experience of my life," she watched as the first blood vessels formed. Over the next two days, she saw the red and white blood cells develop. Finally, the pulsing of the cells told her that the tiny heart had begun to beat.

Sometimes, as when she studied the chick embryo, Sabin worked alone for hours. But frequently, her students worked with her in the laboratory. When a student helped with her research, Florence always shared the credit with the student. If the student had done the bulk of the work, Dr. Sabin put that student's name first when the results were published. This may seem only logical and fair, but it often was, and still is, common to list the senior member of a team first, no matter how meager that member's contribution to the work.

Although she spent most of her time in the laboratory and classroom, Sabin still found time for social activities. She often held dinner parties for groups of students. Many of the doctors brought friends from other professions—lawyers, musicians, or painters. There was always lively conversation over dinner.

Even the meal preparation was an event at Sabin's famous parties. Each guest was assigned a specific task—setting the table, slicing vegetables, washing fruit. In overseeing these tasks, Sabin was, a friend recalled, "as precise as in her laboratory." He described how the guest in charge of turning a steak might be seated in front of the oven with a stopwatch and orders that "at three minutes precisely, not more nor less, the steak was to be turned." After the meal, this amused friend recalled, the dishes were not merely washed, they were boiled as if they had been used in a lab experiment.

As her own family was so far from Baltimore, Florence frequently spent holidays with her friends' families. With her active imagination and warm sympathy, Dr. Sabin became a favorite of the children, bringing gifts of books and organizing taffy pulls.

One hot day, a faculty member fainted during a meeting. He was in no danger, but Sabin realized that his children might hear the news and be frightened. Florence went to their house, where she reassured them. She explained what had happened. Then she made them laugh by falling to the ground in an imitation of fainting. Their anxieties gone, the children played at fainting and recovering until their father came home.

Sabin's friends were like family to her, but she didn't neglect her real family. She maintained her close relationship with her sister, Mary. When she could spare some time, she visited Mary in Denver, where the sisters would go hiking in the mountains. Sometimes Mary accompanied Florence on trips to Europe. Sabin especially liked to visit Germany, where much scientific research was conducted, to learn about the latest laboratory techniques.

Sabin greatly admired German medical studies, and she was very distressed when World War I broke out in 1914. To her, war seemed such a waste. In a lecture she commented, "What a pitiful contrast do the sums we spend on teaching make with the sums we spend on war!" Although Sabin was very absorbed in her work, she tried not to become isolated from the events of the world.

Some of these events involved her directly. As a woman in a mostly male field, Sabin experienced first-hand the struggle of women for equal rights. In the mid-nineteenth century, women had begun to recognize that their roles in society were changing. As more women entered professions, they wanted the same opportunities that men had in education, work, and politics.

Even as late as 1918, women could vote in only

fifteen states. It was clear to women like Florence Sabin that laws and traditions needed to be changed to keep up with the changing roles of women. An organization called the National American Woman Suffrage Association had formed in 1890, and was working to gain the right to vote for all American women. Once they gained the right to vote, women hoped to use their political power to create more equal educational and economic opportunities.

Sabin had not always been a strong supporter of women's rights. Once she had said, "Women get everything they deserve in this life. They needn't think they are discriminated against." As she matured, her experience caused her to change her ideas. A male friend, Dr. Lawrence Kubie, once described her views:

Slowly she saw that for women, as for men, the most difficult part of the struggle for freedom is that struggle for inner freedom which can begin only after external freedoms have been won.

When she could, Florence donated her time to helping women fight for those "external freedoms." During the movement to win voting rights for women, for instance, she wrote many letters of support to legislators. To symbolize her support for the women's movement, she named her first automobile "Susan B.," after the prominent feminist, Susan B. Anthony. In 1920, Sabin celebrated when Congress ratified the nineteenth amendment, which granted women the right to vote in every state of the union.

Florence Sabin's greatest contribution to the women's movement may well have been her public support of women in medicine. In defense of women as research scientists, Florence said, "There are perhaps fewer women working on the scientific side of medicine, but no one would now advocate eliminating the work of a Madame Curie [discoverer of radium] because of a prejudice against the sex of the worker." In another lecture, she exclaimed joyfully: "How glad I am to so affirm my profound faith in the special fitness of women for the medical profession!"

The struggle for women's equality was sometimes a more personal one for Florence Sabin. When Dr. Mall died in 1917, Florence was the logical choice to replace him as head of the Johns Hopkins anatomy department. Instead, a man—a former student of Sabin's—was chosen for the prestigious position. This decision infuriated many of Dr. Sabin's students. But Sabin herself, who had been willing to speak up for other women, was reluctant to fight when her own career was threatened because of her sex. Some students wanted to organize a protest, but Sabin refused to support such action.

When asked if she would stay at Johns Hopkins, Sabin replied, "Of course I'll stay. I have research in progress." Despite the unfair discrimination, Sabin went right on with her work.

Eventually, Dr. Sabin's efforts were rewarded. She was offered a post as chair of the department of histology. This was a less important position than the chair of the anatomy department. But, when she accepted the position, Florence Sabin became the first woman to be appointed a full professor at Johns Hopkins.

As Dr. Sabin's reputation continued to grow, many honorary degrees—seventeen in all—were awarded her. In 1924, Sabin was the first woman to be named president of the American Association of Anatomists. The following year, in 1925, Dr. Sabin became the first woman elected to the National Academy of Sciences.

Also in 1925, Florence was asked to join the Rockefeller Institute for Medical Research in New York City. The decision to leave Johns Hopkins and Baltimore after twenty-five years was hard for her— and it was hard for Johns Hopkins and the city to lose her. When the great teacher and researcher left, the *Baltimore Sun* carried a story about her departure on the front page.

The new position at Rockefeller Institute was purely a research position, involving no teaching. Florence knew that she would miss her students. But she had always longed for the moment when she could devote all her attention to her greatest

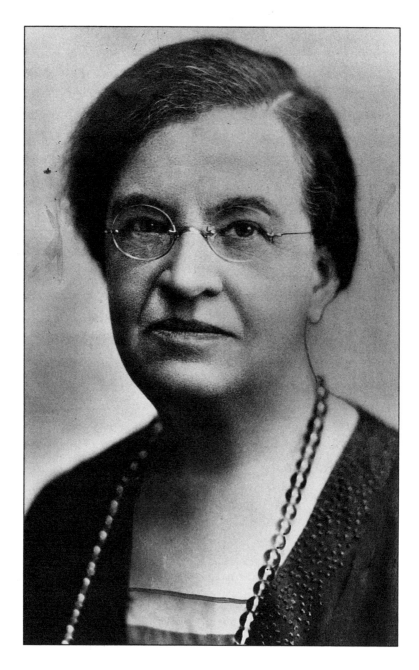

**Florence Sabin, at about the time she left
Baltimore for New York**

passion—research. As she explained to some of her colleagues, "I have ceased to be a professional teacher, but I remain a professional student." Florence Sabin was fifty-one years old.

5

The Importance of the "Littles"

Florence Sabin moved to New York City in the fall of 1925. She was delighted with her new home. She immediately settled into a sunny apartment on the East Side. Florence enjoyed New York's contrasts. She would walk along busy streets shaded by new, tall skyscrapers. Yet, five minutes from the crowded and colorful streets, she could relax among the green woodlands of Central Park. Florence could spend Friday evening watching the most refined opera or concert from plush velvety seats. Then, on Saturday, she could root for the home team, the Brooklyn Dodgers, from the stadium bleachers. She had become a baseball fan in Baltimore, and she continued to follow the game in New York.

Dr. Sabin's greatest pleasure, though, remained

her work. At one dinner party, she ended the late evening by telling her companions that "soon morning will come, and I can again open the door of my beloved laboratory." The Rockefeller Institute, founded in 1901, had become a prestigious center of medical research. Sabin joined the Institute as head of a laboratory for cellular studies. She was the first woman to be invited to full membership at the Institute.

At the Rockefeller Institute, Dr. Sabin was in charge of a group studying tuberculosis (TB). Soon after she arrived at the Institute, she joined the Committee on Medical Research of the National Tuberculosis Association, which was coordinating all tuberculosis research being done in the United States. Her laboratory became part of a nationwide network of hospitals and laboratories working to defeat tuberculosis, an infection of the lungs, which in the early 1900s was the leading cause of death in every age group.

Dr. Sabin wasted no time in assembling her own team of researchers and technicians. Many of these had been students of hers at Johns Hopkins before they followed her to New York. At the Rockefeller Institute, Sabin continued to "pass it on," as Dr. Mall had long ago instructed, sharing both knowledge and credit with her staff. And she continued to demand meticulous, accurate, and original work.

Little was known at that time about how the

tuberculosis infection was transmitted from person to person or about what could be done for those who were ill. Most patients were sent to "sanitariums" to rest for long periods of time. These "rest cures" did not cure but merely stopped the progress of the disease and isolated the patient from people who were well.

In Florence Sabin's laboratory, scientists and technicians studied how tuberculosis affects the blood. The work was tedious. Hours were spent counting the numbers of different types of cells in microscopic blood samples. It took weeks of counting to compile enough information to be useful. This painstaking work took an enormous amount of patience. Once a reporter asked Dr. Sabin if she had made any progress toward finding a cure. "We'll know more about it in fifteen or twenty years," she said.

"Tangible results are not often the reward of a scientist's lifetime," Florence continued. Sometimes, she explained, a scientist "must be content to clear away some of the underbrush, making the way less obstructed for his successors." As Florence Sabin knew, not every experiment leads to a major breakthrough.

Scientific research usually receives little publicity. The most exciting discoveries—a new vaccine or cure, a new surgical technique—will make the news. But such breakthroughs are built on many smaller findings, which usually come from thousands of hours of laboratory work done by hundreds of researchers. The public rarely appreciates the work of these researchers. But without their results, no progress can occur.

Like all researchers, Dr. Sabin followed certain orderly steps. The first job of a researcher, after setting the problem, is to conduct background research to learn what is already known about the problem at hand.

Next, the scientist makes a hypothesis—a prediction about the subject. Then, based on the background information, the researcher designs a study to test the hypothesis. Each step of the experiment is carefully planned. The researcher must try to prepare for anticipated complications.

The researcher then conducts the experiment, repeating, recording, and analyzing each step. Sometimes, the experiment proves that the researcher's hypothesis was correct. But often, the experiment shows that the hypothesis was incorrect.

When the work is done, the researcher summarizes the results, preparing a complete report that includes diagrams and drawings of the experiment. The report is usually published in a scientific journal.

Florence Sabin applied the scientific method carefully. She was very strict about reporting her findings, even when she thought they might be inaccurate.

"The investigator who holds back conclusions until he is absolutely sure, never progresses far," she said. "When I reach certain conclusions, I do not hesitate to publish them, even though, after further study, I may find I was wrong; then I do not hesitate to say that I have changed my mind."

Sabin understood that, for all the excitement of tracking down the truth, there may be only one climactic moment when the researcher finds the central fact she or he has been hunting. After that comes only more of the same, checking and rechecking the procedure and the results.

Though the research conducted by Dr. Sabin's group at the Rockefeller Institute did not lead directly to a cure for tuberculosis, it did contribute to a better understanding of how the tubercle bacillus, the germ that causes tuberculosis, develops and progresses. In the 1940s, partly as a result of the combined national effort, drugs were discovered that were effective in treating most strains of tuberculosis. By the 1960s, tuberculosis was only the eighteenth highest cause of death in the United States, a significant improvement.

No great cure attaches to Florence Sabin's name, and it is hard for those who are not medical scientists to evaluate her contributions to medical research. But Dr. Sabin herself understood the importance of what she called the "littles." She enjoyed working to answer some of the basic questions that underlie the great accomplishments in the sciences.

"Everyone knows that I have no patience with those who think that each new idea is a 'King Strike,'" she said. "I do believe that it is only through cumulative discoveries that greater discoveries take place." Scientists who understood the importance of careful, thorough, and scrupulous work—and its role in supporting the few great breakthroughs—greatly respected and honored the work Dr. Sabin did during this final phase of her research career.

During her career at the Rockefeller Institute, Sabin also took on a non-scientific project: writing Dr. Mall's biography. Florence wanted to pay tribute to her old friend and mentor, but she found the project harder than she expected. The book took her five years to complete. While typing the manuscript, Sabin developed bursitis, an inflammation, in her arm. She later caught pneumonia, and she believed her illness was a direct result of the stress of writing the book. In a letter to Mary, Florence swore never to write another book after *Franklin Paine Mall: The Story of a Mind* was published in 1934.

Florence Sabin also served on the board of directors of many institutions during her years at the Institute. One institution, the University in Exile, was established to relocate and find work for German scholars. Many of these scholars were Jews from Europe who were fleeing the Nazis at the beginning of

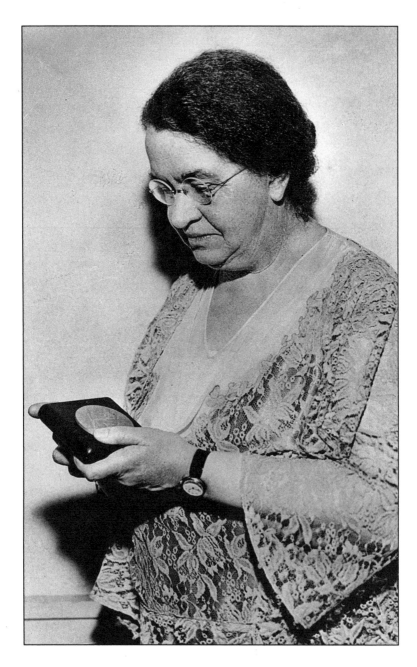

Florence Sabin with the National Achievement
Award from the Chi Omega Sorority, 1932

World War II.

Dr. Sabin was flattered when Albert Einstein, a renowned German-born physicist, personally asked her to find a position for a scientist friend of his. Florence first met Einstein at a dinner party. She was pleased, as she later reported, to discover that Einstein was "utterly simple, as all great thinkers are." In a letter to her sister, Mary, she described the prominent physicist as a man whose "laugh rings out and makes everyone around him happy."

Florence and Mary still wrote regularly to each other and pledged to make their retirement home together. When Mary retired from teaching in 1931, she tried to persuade Florence to leave the Institute and return to Denver with her. But at that time, Florence Sabin was enjoying her research too much to retire. She passed her sixty-fifth birthday, the age at which most people retire, and kept right on working.

In 1938, when Florence was sixty-seven, she did retire. Rockefeller Institute had decided to enforce a mandatory retirement age. Dr. Sabin was sorry to leave, but she understood the need to provide younger workers with research opportunities. Her fulfilling research career was over.

Sabin's friends and colleagues planned a surprise party for her retirement dinner. They gathered at the Rainbow Room, located on the top floor of Rockefeller Center. Florence suspected nothing when a few friends invited her out for dinner. Even when they reached the party, at first she thought it was just a coincidence that so many of her friends were there. She was too modest to think that the grand dinner had been prepared in her honor.

After the dinner, Dr. Sabin talked about her years as a researcher. Medical science had seen many changes in the time since Sabin had graduated from medical school. After describing her recent work, she concluded, "The most interesting thing about it all is that in the last few weeks I have discovered that everything I have been doing in these last few years is all wrong."

"She went on to say," one guest remembered, "why this did not matter, why the negative results of science pave the way for the positive findings of others, and how the important thing in the end is the progress of knowledge and not which individual is the relay runner who for a brief span carries the torch."

6

A Very Short Retirement

At first, Florence enjoyed retirement. She and Mary decorated their apartment in Denver with Persian and Turkish rugs. The sisters went hiking together and took a pleasant trip to Alaska. In addition to leisure activities, there was always scientific work that Florence could do. She did some cellular research at the University of Colorado, wrote papers, gave lectures, went to meetings, and joined the board of directors at Denver's Children's Hospital. She often visited the Rockefeller Institute, where she was welcome to work at any time, as an honored guest.

During these early years of her retirement, Sabin had a personal bookplate designed with a picture of a microscope and a translated quote from the great Italian renaissance artist and scientist Leonardo da Vinci.

It read, "Thou, O God, dost sell unto us all good things at the price of labour." Sabin believed in hard work, and she was growing bored with retirement. She found it hard to adjust to a life where little was expected of her. She expected more of herself.

But her restlessness was soon to end. It was 1944, and the country was shifting gears. People all across the nation were longing for an end to World War II, and were making plans in anticipation of the changes peace would bring.

In Colorado, Governor John Vivian was forming a planning commission to help the state move into the post-war era. A female reporter challenged the governor when she learned that there were no women appointed to the commission. She suggested that he appoint Florence Sabin to head the subcommittee on health. The governor agreed. He thought it was unlikely that a retired doctor in her seventies would cause him any trouble.

When Governor Vivian asked if she would head the health subcommittee, Dr. Sabin agreed. Forty-four years after receiving her medical degree, she enthusiastically began to practice a kind of medicine she had never tried before.

Although the public health field was new to Florence Sabin, it had been of concern to governments since the earliest times. Wherever people established communities, they needed methods of waste disposal, disease control, and water purification.

In the 1800s, public health problems increased as more and more people began to move to cities. Epidemics of contagious diseases like smallpox and typhoid were continual problems in crowded, dirty American cities. In desperation, private groups of social reformers established programs to improve the cleanliness, or sanitation, of water, streets, food, and medical facilities. Soon, state and local governments began to create public agencies to regulate health. In 1878, the federal government began a health service for merchant sailors. This agency eventually grew to serve all Americans and was renamed the United States Public Health Service in 1912.

By the 1940s, most states had their own agencies to control and prevent disease, promote sanitary food and water, and provide community health services. The agencies of different states varied in effectiveness.

Florence Sabin's job was to look into the laws and practices of the state and community agencies of Colorado. She would evaluate how they were affecting people's health. Then, she could help bring about whatever changes were necessary to improve the health of the citizens of Colorado.

The public health laws then in effect in Colorado had been passed in 1876. Dr. Sabin saw that they clearly needed updating. In order to revise those laws, she would draw upon the skills she had developed during forty years of teaching and research. She would use her training in research to help her get at the facts she needed. Her medical training would be useful for understanding the implications for people's health. The teaching skills she had acquired would help her educate the public about what she had learned. And her experience in organizing people into an effective working group would help her rally the support she needed.

Dr. Sabin's research and teaching skills would be a great help, but she sensed that they would not be enough. All her life, Florence had kept a low profile, even as she received numerous awards and honors for her work. But in this new job, she knew she would need to seek out publicity. She would not accomplish anything unless she spoke out and took some bold political actions.

In the eighth decade of her life, Florence Sabin changed her quiet habits and became an outspoken advocate for public health. She astonished the elected officials of Colorado when she turned out to have a knack for effective politics.

One of Sabin's first steps as a public health worker was to ask the American Public Health Association to make a survey of the health conditions in Colorado. Dr. Carl Buck, from the Association, studied the situation and gave Sabin his report in January of 1946. She called the report "masterly." The author,

Sabin reported, had "studied the vital statistics of the State Health Division." He had "analyzed and arranged the data until they told a vivid story of the state's health deficiencies."

The report held startling news: thirty-four states and the District of Columbia had better records than Colorado in preventing deaths from controllable diseases. And only four of Colorado's sixty-three counties had full-time health services. The report showed that, between 1940 and 1944, 14,552 Coloradans had died from "preventable or controllable diseases."

The report also analyzed the reasons for Colorado's poor health conditions. Colorado was giving its Division of Public Health less than ten cents per person to protect the health of its citizens. Serious diseases like tuberculosis went undiagnosed and untreated, and there weren't enough hospital beds for the sick people in the state.

To make matters worse, the State Health Division was poorly run, and the local health authorities that regulated health in individual towns and counties were even worse. Most were not taking commonplace precautions to protect the health of their citizens. Milk was not regulated or inspected. Barely half the communities had adequate, pollution-free water supplies. Only sixteen percent of the communities had modern sewage systems. Nearly half had no system for purifying sewage before it was dumped into streams to pollute irrigation waters and contaminate crops.

Dr. Sabin realized that many of Colorado's health problems stemmed from the beef and dairy industries—two of the state's biggest money-makers. The state had no effective control of the milk supply. It had no authority to regulate dairy herds or milk production. As a result, there was no statewide provision for the purification, or pasteurization, of milk. In Colorado, the motto was "cattle is king." The powerful cattle industry had prevented the state from taking effective preventive measures against brucellosis, a disease carried by almost half the state's cattle. This disease caused serious illness in people who ate meat or drank milk from sick cows.

The beef and dairy industries were so important to the state and national economy that the industries had great control over any measures that might affect them. For years, they had been able to prevent the state from regulating their products.

Dr. Sabin wasted no time in taking action. She immediately had copies of Dr. Buck's report circulated. "We heard that the Buck Report was going to be put in a desk drawer and locked up," she remembered later, "so what we did was have a thousand copies struck off. It's hard to get a thousand copies into a desk drawer. And we distributed them."

Sabin then gathered her forces. She invited groups of Colorado's leaders in medicine, finance, public affairs and eventually, even the cattlemen themselves to a series of dinners at Denver's famous Brown's Palace Hotel. Her goal was to learn more about Colorado's health situation, to educate others and stimulate their interest, and to enlist support for the changes she knew were needed.

After each meal, Dr. Sabin explained her purpose and gave a brief but compelling description of the terrible health conditions in Colorado. Following her summary, Dr. Sabin encouraged her guests to talk and trade ideas. People from the state civil service commission, for instance, talked about improving staffing at the health departments. People from medical and public health groups traded information and ideas about the distressing tuberculosis situation. Sanitary engineers discussed the need for adequate sewage disposal.

Some of Dr. Sabin's guests, such as former Colorado State Senator Price Briscoe, were easily recruited. Until he met Florence Sabin, Briscoe said, "I was just an ex-Senator minding my own business and running a gold mine." Before Senator Briscoe knew what was happening, he had agreed to work on a committee. "And I'm not the only one," the senator said. "Dr. Sabin has scores of people just like me, who've caught the torch for something that nobody ever could have gotten us excited about before."

Not all of Dr. Sabin's guests "caught the torch" so

easily. The meat and dairy industries viewed her as a threat—most of Sabin's proposed measures would cost them a great deal of money.

When Florence Sabin finally had the information and resources she needed, she and her supporters began to take action. The health committee drafted a series of bills to present to the state legislature. The bills dealt with a wide range of issues: they provided funding for new hospitals, and better care for tuberculosis patients. And they established measures to curtail the spread of brucellosis among cattle. Sabin knew that the future health of the people of Colorado depended on the passage of this legislation, which came to be known as the "Sabin bills."

Dr. Sabin realized that she could not count on the legislators, many of whom depended on the financial support of uncooperative cattle industries, to pass her bills. She needed to gather massive public support. "The winning of popular support for the program was crucial to its success," Sabin reported later. "Since this was a state program, popular education was started in the counties."

Florence Sabin took her campaign straight to the people. In the election of 1946, citizens of Colorado would vote for governor and for the members of their state legislature. This new legislature would vote on the Sabin bills, and, if the bills passed, the new governor would put the reforms into practice. Sabin had to convince the voters to make health conditions an important campaign issue.

For the first time in her life, Florence Sabin was engaged in medical work that would have an immediate effect on the public's health. Using the slogan, "Health to Match Our Mountains," she traveled around the state, spreading the word wherever she could find an audience. During the months, weeks, and days before the election, Florence Sabin spoke two or three times a day, in cities and towns throughout Colorado.

Dr. Sabin's method of educating the public was simple. She merely guided the voters through the same steps she herself had taken: learning the truth about existing health conditions, deciding which conditions must be changed, then deciding how to change those conditions.

Sabin's approach was remarkably similar to the philosophy she had applied as a teacher. She presented the material, leaving the citizens to act. Again, her technique proved effective.

Sabin's energy for her campaign seemed without limits. She traveled hundreds of miles across the mountains to bring her message to people in remote rural towns. Even blizzards did not keep her from arriving at her destination. She addressed anyone who would listen, including parent-teacher associations, medical associations, or farmers' groups.

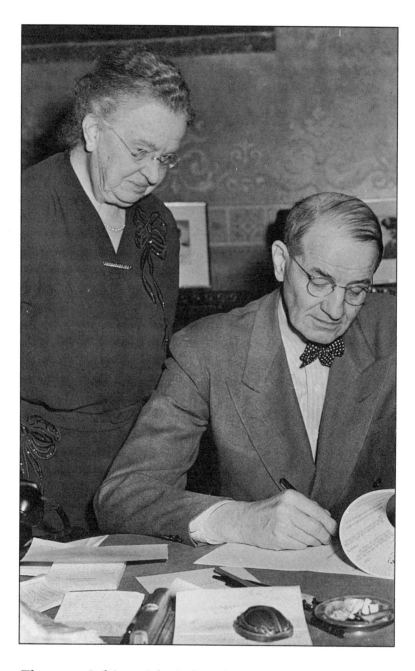

Florence Sabin with Colorado Governor Lee Knous

Soon, Florence's persistence began to pay off. As the election drew near, health became a central issue in the campaign. Each politician was questioned about his position on the Sabin bills; each candidate was forced to take a stand.

As it turned out, every legislator who had spoken against the Sabin program was defeated in the election of 1946. Long-standing officials who had ignored the Sabin bills lost to newcomers who had supported the measures.

Governor Vivian, the very man who had appointed Florence Sabin to head the health subcommittee, had in the end opposed her. He was defeated by a candidate who had applauded the Sabin bills at every opportunity. "When it comes to those bills. . . there isn't a man in the legislature who wants to tangle with her," said the new governor, Lee Knous. "She's an atom bomb."

7

Defending Denver's Health

Most of the new legislators agreed with the governor's assessment. "We all knew in advance that this time we had to pass the health bills," said one newly elected official. And most of the Sabin bills did pass in the next legislative session. Dr. Sabin worked directly with the lawmakers and was in the meeting chambers during all debates. Only the "cow bill," which provided for control of brucellosis, did not pass. The cattlemen had convinced their legislators that such a bill would prove too costly.

But defeat only revived Sabin's efforts. She applied a philosophy she had used during her medical research: "Defeat is often the first step toward improvement." Once again she made dinner reservations at Brown's Palace Hotel, and she invited representatives of the cattle industry.

Dr. Sabin explained to the industry representatives that healthier cows would actually increase their profits. She presented studies showing that an infected cow produced far less milk than a healthy cow. Calves often died from disease, another costly loss for the industry. She demonstrated that healthier cows would increase the industry's long-term production of both milk and meat.

Florence Sabin convinced the businessmen that healthy cows would earn more money for them than sick cows would. They agreed to remove their opposition to the "cow bills." When the legislation was brought up in the legislature again, it passed.

In a speech to the Western Branch of the American Public Health Association in 1947, Florence Sabin summed up what she had learned from the experience:

> No wonder Coloradans walk on air and talk of health to match their mountains! They have won the decisive battles of their campaign and now have only to get on with the business of public health in Colorado.

Sabin was triumphant. The Division of Health hadn't even had a phone number before, she said. "Now, there are eight departments offering a full quota of health services." The Sabin bills attracted qualified health officials by increasing salaries and improving employment conditions. They granted health authorities the right to inspect water supplies, sewage disposal, milk and meat supplies, and vegetables.

But Florence Sabin knew that her work was far from over. Some Colorado cities, such as Denver, were exempt from the new state laws. Many of her newly won reforms would have little effect in those cities.

In 1947, Dr. Sabin accepted an appointment to chair Denver's Interim Board of Health and Hospitals. She would not accept a salary for this position, insisting instead that the money be donated to the University of Colorado School of Medicine.

Once again, Sabin's investigations detected serious health problems. The city had no schedule of garbage collection. Alleys were strewn with trash. Rats abounded. Restaurants were not inspected. Tuberculosis rates were high.

Just as she had done before, Dr. Sabin made health a central campaign issue—this time in a mayoral election. And again, the outspoken health candidate won—by more votes than all four other candidates combined. Dr. Sabin then designed, planned, and initiated a series of successful programs that brought about significant improvements in the health of Denver's residents. She instituted a free x-ray program to diagnose tuberculosis in early,

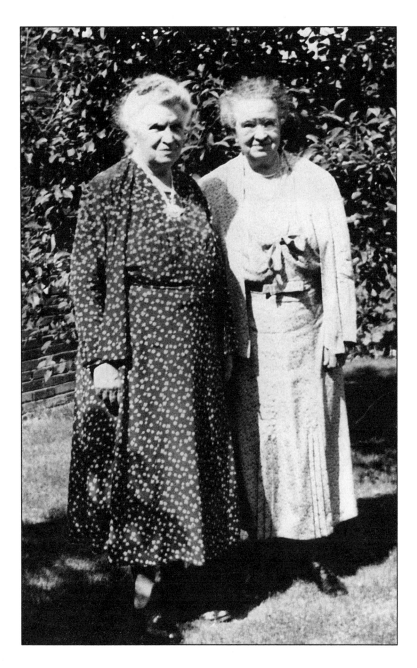

**Florence Sabin (right) with her sister Mary,
in Denver**

treatable stages. Within two years, Denver's tuberculosis death rate was cut in half.

One day in 1949, Dr. Sabin was moving about with a mobile x-ray unit, encouraging people to have free x-rays as part of the program against tuberculosis. A reporter approached and asked the elderly doctor how she could keep going—she was getting close to eighty, after all!

She answered:

Labor. Labor is not a grinding ordeal to which one is driven by the whip of necessity. It's a privilege. Whether work means digging ditches, driving a car, or working for world understanding, it will keep you healthy and young if you work with enjoyment. It's resistance to work—not work itself—that ages people.

8

Teacher, Scientist, Humanitarian

Her work in Denver was Florence Sabin's final public health victory. In 1952, she retired for good. She decided to retire because Mary's health was failing, and she wanted to care for her sister. Some time later, Florence made the difficult decision to commit her sister to professional care in a nursing home.

Although she was in failing health herself, Florence Sabin continued in her "real" retirement to be interested in public and medical issues, and she read and corresponded widely. In 1952, for instance, she urged Colorado to follow California's lead in fighting air pollution. That same year, the American Association of University Women established a Florence R. Sabin fellowship to honor those who had made important contributions in public health. The eighty-year-old Dr. Sabin was also given the Elizabeth Blackwell Citation and the University of Colorado's Distinguished Service Award.

In October of 1953, Florence Sabin was thrilled when "her" Brooklyn Dodgers captured the National League pennant. She cheered them enthusiastically as they took on the New York Yankees in the World Series. She watched the fourth World Series game on her television set, with a nurse who was staying at her home, monitoring her health. When it came time for the traditional seventh-inning stretch, the nurse helped Florence to her feet. She stood momentarily, then collapsed. Florence Sabin was dead of a heart attack at the age of eighty-one.

* * *

Florence Sabin's contributions spanned half a century. As a scientist, Dr. Sabin contributed to early knowledge of the body's cells and how they work. Later, she developed more complex investigations and studied the role of human cells in fighting disease. Her exacting work was an important resource for scientists who came after her.

Sabin's dedication to her work was unselfish. For years, she taught at Johns Hopkins, taking hours from her own work to supervise students in the laboratory. Many of Dr. Sabin's students later became prominent researchers. In 1951, her ability as a teacher was

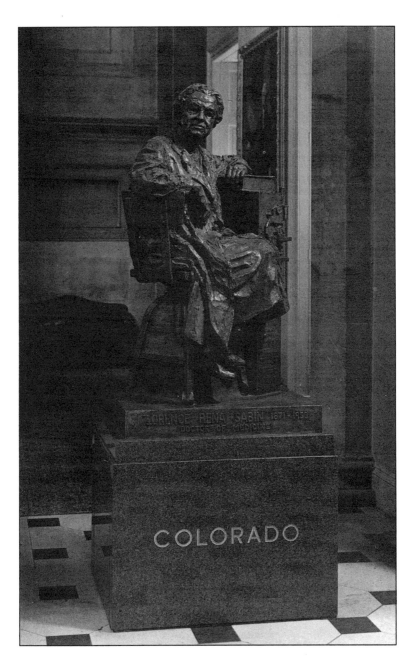

A tribute to Dr. Florence Sabin, Statuary Hall,
Washington, D.C.

recognized when the University of Colorado dedicated the new Florence R. Sabin Building for Research in Cellular Biology. "For Dr. Sabin, the ideal of great teaching is stimulation of the student to the love and pursuit of knowledge," said the dedication speaker, Dr. Grover F. Powers. "The impact of her teaching upon pupils is to inculcate a love of scholarship, a high regard for learning, a fostering of the spirit of inquiring and of intellectual curiosity."

Florence Sabin's devotion to students and to science did not end with her death. In her will, she left several hundred thousand dollars to the University of Colorado School of Medicine to be used to support educational programs and research.

Dr. Sabin never lost her own spirit of intellectual curiosity. When her career as a researcher and teacher was over, she was ready to delve into a new field. At a time when most people retire, Florence worked harder than ever, launching a tireless campaign to improve the health of the people of Colorado.

When Florence Sabin died, the *Rocky Mountain News* quoted the mayor of Denver, Quigg Newton, who said: "She was learned, she was wise, she was humble. She loved the world and every creature in it." An article in the *Denver Post* called Dr. Sabin the "First Lady of American Science," a title she richly deserved.

For Further Reading

Readers who want to find out more about the life of Florence Sabin may be interested in these books:

- *Women and Science* by Valjean McLenighan. Florence Sabin is one of six women discussed in this book (Raintree, 1979).

- *Probing the Unknown: The Story of Dr. Florence Sabin* by Mary Kay Phelan (Crowell, Women of America series, 1969).

- *Florence Sabin: Medical Researcher* by Janet Kronstadt (Chelsea House, American Women of Achievement series, 1990).

- *Women Pioneers of Science* by Louis Haber. Discusses Florence Sabin's life and work in a chapter titled "Public Health Physician" (Harcourt Brace, 1979).

Readers looking for information on other famous women in science may want to read:

- *Nobel Prize Women in Science: Their Lives, Struggles and Momentous Discoveries* by Sharon McGrayne Bertsch (Birch Lane Press/Carol Publishing Group, 1992).

Index

References to photographs are listed in *italic, **boldface*** type.